Revised edition depicting the 2nd knee replacement
"The same, but different"

Total Knee & Hip Replacement

What you need to know!

Day by day Account of One Man's Journey Plus Interviews with people who've made the journey from start to finish

DISCLAIMER

This book and its contents is for information purposes only and not meant to impart medical advice or give instructions of a medical nature. Any suggestions given here, are suggestions only and not meant to be taken as medical advice. When in deciding upon or adopting a procedure of any medical nature make sure to consult your primary care doctor or a physician before making any decision to do so. The author Roger Breternitz, is not a medical doctor or connected with the medical field in any way and only a first hand observer/patient in the procedure of knee replacement, and assumes no liability in the publishing of this book or the suggestions given therein along with A Winners Way and Vector Studios. None of the people interviewed are medical doctors, in the medical field or to be construed as same, and are only giving their accounts of their experiences as they happened and not to be taken as medical recommendations in any way.

ISBN-13:978-1530728558
ISBN-10:153072855X
LCCN:2016905261

Cover - Logo Design & Published by
Roger W. Breternitz CCht.
&
Vector Studios®
very sound investment

Laguna Niguel Ca.

Website: www.awinnersway.com
Website: www.vectorstudios.com

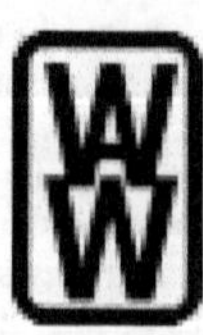

Total Knee & Hip Replacement

What you need to know!

A Day-By-Day Account
of the experience, feelings, reactions and overview that are omitted from the brochures and manuals

A MUST READ, FOR EVERY POTENTIAL PATIENT

By Roger W. Breterntiz CCht.

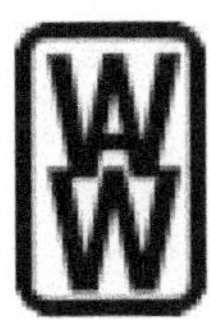

Table of Contents

FORWARD

Every time you think about going out on that "Limb of the unknown, Edge of the Universe, Uncharted waters", or whatever it is that you're not sure of, you wish that there was someone you could ask about this big question mark. Someone that doesn't stand to profit from, or gain from their "Advice".

That is what this book is all about. It's written with as little bias as possible, and just states the facts. If the facts say, "This hospital did a great job" then I mention it, but they're not hiring me to write this. I felt compelled to write this because if one person reads it and gains a little insight into what they're ***about*** to experience, then maybe I've helped in them making a decision. If I have possibly helped hasten their path to recovery, maybe make things a little better for them or prevented them from going down a wrong path, this is a good thing, and it will come back to me in positive ways that will never end.

Because knee and hip replacements are very much alike, in that people go through much of the same challenges in rehabilitation, pain management, and recovery, you can basically read this book from either vantage point of hip or knee replacement.

Hopefully you can learn from some of my

mistakes, like getting off pain killers, and physical therapy mistakes, maybe even arriving at the "To do – Not to do" decision, which is the biggest fork in the road before any of this all begins to take place.

When you read the publications and brochures about knee & hip replacements, talk to the doctors, and even friends who have had it done, there's a lot they don't tell you, even more they forgot to tell you, and the only way you will ever learn what it's really like, is to do it, then you go back to them and say, "Why didn't you tell me about xxx?

So on your adventure to get this done before you are "To old", I wish you the best of luck, while hoping that luck has nothing to do with the actual process of the operation. If what you learn here in these pages helps you make a better and more informed decision, then I've done a good thing, best of "Luck", hoping luck has nothing to do with it.

AUTHOR'S NOTE:
Since we remember half of what we see, a quarter of what we hear and less than that, of what we read, I have chose to mention sections of information several times in different places to help instill that information in your conscious mind so you will remember it. So if you think you've already read something, you probably have.

Chapter 1
Why do you want a total knee or hip replacement?

All our lives we have wants and needs, and hopeful most of the times those two line up. However, for some people they very rarely line up. When they don't line up, meaning the things they need and the things they want, That's when you've got a problem.

So in this case you need to stake stock of "This is what I want, but this is what I need. Maybe you don't really need a new knee or hip just yet, but I want one because of certain factors. What would be those factors?

1. I want to do it before I get "Too old". Everybody has a reference point as to many things and the term "Too old" is one of them. You can go along just as you are now with some marginal pain but you know sooner or later you're going to have to get this "Thing" done, and that's a good point. Older people react differently to the drugs and anesthetics they are given, their rate of healing is much slower, recovery time is much longer.

2. I want to do it because I want to be as good at "MY" sport as it "Use to be". This was my reason in wanting to get a new knee, in addition to the fact

I had absolutely no cartilage on the right side of my knee and I was "Knock kneed" with my joint in close to the center of my body.
Tennis was more than a "Big deal" to me. I played in a major university for 2 years, then came to California where I established a teaching concern called "Learn Tennis" and since my degree was in education, I began to use what I learned to formulate several teaching methods I still use today and people were very satisfied saying they really improved or they felt like they really learned something. And of course I played and won several tournaments, and I could be pretty competitive. That was when I was 35-55. I was also a ski instructor at one of the local mountains in Big Bear California, and if tennis didn't trash my cartilage, ski instruction each weekend, really did it for me. Suddenly I began to feel a new level of pain coming from my right knee, but I could still move to the tennis ball, and my doctor told me to give up playing singles and stick to doubles, which I did for the next 10 years. Now my knee is down to bone on bone, I could barely take 2 steps toward the ball, and I have to play with lower level players to keep from being embarrassed. So 2 hours before playing I take 2 Advil jells, and that helps the pain and allows me to half run half hobble to balls more than a couple of steps away from my location. Finally when I turned 71, one day I was dragging myself around the court and I came to the epiphany "That's it, got to get a new

knee." I could still walk fine, not too much pain, but I was a tennis pro who couldn't keep up with my students because I just could not get to the ball. So for me, is was a "Want" thing as well as a "Need" thing. Most of the people I talk to who have had the knee or hip replacement, say much the same thing, "I should have had it done years ago".

So, the point of this chapter is, consider very carefully why you want…or need…a knee or hip replacement. If it falls in the "Need" department, then get it done, start talking to your doctor immediately, call your insurance company, and see what they will authorize and pay for, what your co-pay will be in a ballpark figure. Then just take the first step to getting it done, you WILL be better off for it. Usually people who are just thinking about getting it done, but don't need it right now will wait until it graduates to the "Need" category, then *they* are the people who say they should have had it done years ago.

If it falls into the "Want" department, then at least you are not forced to get the operation, it's something that you want to do. When you consider the big picture, it is sometimes better to undergo the procedure and all of its negatives when *you* choose the time and place, rather than your knee or hip, or the pain chooses for you. You are in more control and there is a lot to be said for that.
In considering putting it off, there is the school of

thought that says, “You’re not getting any younger”, and everything is tougher on you the older you get.

As we get older we don’t have the same abilities to mend like we used to. Our body cells don’t seem to reproduce as fast as they use to, not to mention our immune system is not as strong as it was when we were younger, but then we didn’t need a “New knee or hip” when we were younger.

Whatever your thinking is, you may want to subscribe to my mantra of life…”Just do it.”

Chapter 2
Steps you will go through

Consultation. First of all you will have a consultation with your primary doctor, who will then make a referral appointment with your surgeon. As I previously stated just because my health coverage was Kaiser, they're not paying me to write this, I'm just stating it as a fact. They are very professional, the staff is of the highest level, and the doctor who performed my surgery was very well known as one of the top knee/hip surgeons, not only within Kaiser, but by the entire medical community in Orange County California. He did a masterful job, and you can hardly even see the scar. There, that's the last you'll hear about who did my knee replacement and how great a job it was.

Health Screening. After this initial consultation with your surgeon you will be scheduled for a health screening to determine if you are a healthy enough person to stand the rigors of the surgery and anesthetic along with the pain medication.

Surgery? Then you will be scheduled for surgery, or NOT! You may have to wait as much as 3 months, because your doctor has that much of a waiting list. When you do get your surgery date, it's time for you to start your PRE-surgery exercise. You need to build up your leg muscles to a higher level than they are right now, because you won't be using them anywhere close to the level you were before. You'll be weak in that area for a long time and physical therapy will help you get back that original strength. However; if you can start out with a strong physical condition, you're way ahead of the game. You can hire a professional physical therapist or do your own therapy if you have a good work ethic, but much more about that in future chapters.

This PT is very important to your life with your new knee or hip. Scar tissue forms in the area of the surgery and must be broken up, and this is *painful*, even on the pain killers they will give you, but it must be done. The two major hurdles you will encounter are getting the degree of flexibility to bending your knee or your hip in the directions necessary to achieve maximum flexibility. As far as your knee, in this case it is bringing your ankle back up to your thigh so that the angle of your lower leg and upper leg is at least 140 degrees. Your therapist will measure this with a plastic protractor so it's not just a general ballpark figure. This *must* achieved in the first 2 months while the scar tissue is workable. Like my therapist told me as he was forcing my lower leg back toward the thigh,(and causing me an immense amount of pain) "You can hate me know or hate me later (for not doing it). Meaning if you don't get the flexibility now while the scar tissue is workable, you will not

have the flexibility for the rest of your life. All that money, pain, and, discomfort you've experienced will be for naught!
If you learn anything from this book learn that!

Preparation for surgery

First of all depending upon your present weight, if you are over weight you should plan on losing as much as necessary to get down to your correct weight, because you're not going to be doing a lot of calorie burning activities while getting back to the life you're use to. It is also a good idea to build yourself up by going to the gym and doing some strengthening exercises or lifting a few moderate weights, because you will be focusing more on getting the angular degree of flexibility between your upper and lower leg. Then later you will be doing the strengthening exercises to restore your entire leg to its original capability. So, it would be good if you had built up the muscles around your knee or hip to begin with before hand.

Medications

You will be given specific instructions on which medications to stop, and when to stop them in relation to your day of surgery. These instructions are vey important because they regulate your blood clotting ability, blood pressure, and more. If you are taking dietary supplements these should be stopped two weeks before the operation, but consult your physician to make sure.

Smoking, alcohol and drugs

Stop smoking prior to surgery, since it's a proven fact that smoking is bad for your lungs and general well being, you want to be in the best condition possible before your surgery.
Alcohol: DO NOT use alcohol 2 weeks before surgery. It has adverse effect on the meds you will be given, both painkillers, and antibiotics.
Drugs: Never use controlled substances or related drugs before any surgery.

Night before surgery

Do not eat or drink anything after midnight.

The night before surgery you will use the sterilization packed you've been given to wipe your entire body (after shower) with a special astringent to kill any bacteria and help eliminate the possibility of infection. Much of what is done before, during, and after the operation focuses on that specific theme. Infection is your worst enemy, it can cause you a world of hurt, and setback.

Morning before surgery

Once again (without showering) you will use the second packet given you to wipe your entire body in the manner described in the instructions. This gives further protection against infection. Brush your teeth after eating or before leaving home. Give yourself plenty of time to arrive.

Don't wear makeup, body lotion, or deodorant.
Wear loose clothing easily removable, preferably no belts, and the like. Wear slippers, or slip-on sneakers or shoes.
Bring only enough money to cover your co-pay, your ID, leave wallet at home, don't bring any valuables, cell phones, credit cards, keys or jewelry, you won't need them. It would be good to bring a book because there probably will be some slack time.

Preparing your home

One of the first things you need to do is to remove all throw rugs, floor rugs, and any thing that could be considered a hindrance to someone using a walker, crutches, or cane. That is how you're going to start out, using a walker until you get enough strength and resistance to pain to start using crutches or a cane.

It's all about baby steps in the beginning, then putting more weight on the leg in question, and each week or day (depending upon your progress) you are able to put more and more weight on the leg, until you no longer need a cane. This will take some time, and be very careful not to rush things.

Take it slow, be very deliberate in your movements and actions, and let people help you. I can't imagine going through an operation like this without securing someone to help you, and be with you on a 24/7 basis, or at least 10 hours out of the day, in the daylight hours.

Here's a bit of advice. When you are finally out of the house, walking and driving, remember one thing. STUFF HAPPENS, and you don't want it to happen to you! So, always be vigilant, be aware of your surroundings, and the people / animals / vehicles / bicycles / skateboards/ roller-skaters / and anyone else in your immediate vicinity. If they look like they're not in control of their pets, kids, cars, or themselves…*stay away from them*!

Commit this to memory

LIVE IS NOT A VIDEO TAPE, THERE IS NO REWIND, NO REPLAY!

Chapter 3
Equipment you will need

Walker

This is a device with wheels in front and rubber feet in the back. You put both hands on the handles, rest most of your weight on those handles and put a small amount of weight on the leg with your new knee or hip and walk forward. Each day you walk a little further, putting more weight on that particular leg. Finally you will be able to switch to a cane to bare most of the weight instead of your leg. Then you begin to ease into putting more pressure on that knee or hip joint and less pressure on the cane.

Bamboo cane

The best cane I found was one of fire hardened bamboo with the standard crook at the top. Trouble with that one is you would most likely need to saw it off to be just the right height in relation to your hand position.

Using a cane effectively, is not as easy as it sounds. First of all the cane has to be just the right height from the ground for you to lock your elbow stiffly making your upper and lower arm as straight as possible, and then push it firmly up against your hip to keep it there as you put all your weight on it. Now you are using it to support the weight that your leg with your new knee or hip, should be taking. With each step the cane is positioned like it is almost attached to the leg in question. As the leg moves, so does the cane. As the knee or hip gets better and more healed, you can put less weight on the cane and more weight on the side of your body in question.

In my case, after the 4th day, I didn't need the cane any more, but on my therapy walks around the block where I live, I would *always* take the cane with me anyway as defense against unruly dogs not kept in check by their careless owners, or unruly kids not kept in check by their careless parents. One little brat on a skateboard could take you out in a heartbeat, and a $45,000 knee or hip replacement is wiped away. The mother says, "Oh I'm so sorry, I didn't realize my little boy was coming down the sidewalk on his new skate board he hasn't really learned how to ride YET! Don't count on her to pay your hospital bill to set you right again! No rewind – no replay!

Aluminum adjustable cane

These are the kind that pharmacies sell for around $40 and some of them have actually have 3 rubber feet so they will stand up on their own if you let go of them. The best feature of these canes is they are adjustable to any height you need, and some of them actually collapse to 3 sections for easy

transportation when not in use. My suggestion is to

never cut costs when purchasing something to help you in a medical situation. You are going to spend a considerable amount of money to get this done, buy equipment you can trust.

Ice flow/pac machine

This delivers a flow of cold water to a bladder which you adhere to your knee or hip with a series of Velcro bands. It keeps the area cold better than an ice pack and intern keeps the swelling down. You fill it with ice water and it does a great job to reducing inflammation.

Money Saving Tip for flow pack machine

Get some medium size water bottles, fill them up and put in the freezer. You can re-use them over and over again like several big ice cubes that are re-freezable. Put them in the freezer at night and they're ready in the AM. Get 8 of them and keep recycling them 4 at a time if you want to use the icing machine for a full day. Otherwise you will be buying a LOT of ice.

Compression Socks

These knee length support socks prevent a blood clot in your lower leg or calf area. If this happens (in addition to being dangerous to your health) it will complicate your life like you cannot imagine! You'll need to wear them for about 6 to 8 weeks, and they can be hard to get on when you have other standard length socks on to keep your toes warm (they have no toe covering). Still they are very important to your wellbeing so just get use to wearing them. After about 5 weeks you can stop their use and go back to regular socks.

Chapter 4

My account of the procedure and related events

August 5, 2015
Initial consultation with my surgeon

I met with my "Potential" surgeon and we discussed my desire to get a total knee replacement. The questions that were asked were,
Q. How much pain I was in at the time.
A: Only when I try to make quick movements on the tennis court, or try to walk for a longer distance that a mile.

Q. What am I doing to help the pain?
A: Taking an anti-inflammatory like Advil. Did I realize that prolonged usage of this would be detrimental for my stomach and liver? I said I only took it before I played tennis or anticipated a long walking situation.

Q. Did I realize that the total knee replacement would improve my ability to move but never give me back my original movement or mobility.
A. Yes I did, and would welcome any improvement.

Q. Did I realize that I would be incapacitated for a period of 3 to 4 weeks, and would need someone to take care of me for that time.

A. Yes, I was lucky enough to have my wife who had just retired from her nursing position to help me.

Q. Was I allergic to any drugs, pain killers, and medicines?

A. No, I could take most any antibiotics, pain killers etc.

Q. What kind of environment did I live in as far as up stairs / down stairs bedrooms.

A. My bedrooms are up stairs, but I didn't see a problem with it.

I was scheduled for X-rays and had them taken that day.

After the reading of the X-rays the surgeon said I was a good candidate for the surgery and would put me on a list of waiting patients. Because the list was so long, it may take 3 months to be scheduled. The hospital would call me when they were able to schedule me for the surgery.

Nov. 4, 2015

Hospital calls and informs me they have scheduled me for surgery on Dec. 22, 2015. I will stay in the hospital for 2 days and come home on Dec. 24,

2015, Christmas Eve. I did not argue about it after waiting this long to get the surgery date, so be it!

Nov. 12, 2015

Evaluation & screening for surgery

A doctor for the hospital meets with me to do heart EKG monitoring, and screening of my general health conditions, take blood pressure, blood samples and ask many of the same questions that I answered on the screening form given me a week ago. It was determined that I was a good candidate for the procedure, and I was scheduled to meet with my surgeon again.

Dec. 2, 2015

Pre-surgery orientation

This was a meeting of all of the people who had applied to get a knee/hip replacement. Most of them above the age of 70 like me. A physical therapist gets up in front of the room as gives a 2 hour lecture on all of the aspects of the procedure, what to expect, how long therapy will take and many other interesting factors that people will need to know about their up coming operation. He finishes up with a question/answer session that lasts another half hour.

Dec. 8, 2015

Meeting with my surgeon

We discussed the procedure, all of the aspects and repercussions therein. He showed my by the use of a plastic model of the knee and tendons, how the operation would take place, and in quite detail gave me a run down of the entire procedure. He was a very personable and forth coming individual and I felt very comfortable with him in charge of my procedure.

He told me that the hospital has only 2 dedicated rooms for total knee & hip replacement and all they do in those dedicated rooms is tare those types operations. No other kinds of procedures of operations. They have two teams consisting of one surgeon, anesthesiologist, and 2 support techs. All they do is knee & hip replacements, and they've done thousands. They know every move, every aspect, and they work like clockwork, to insure total success, and protect against infection. I felt very secure in their care and left with a very positive feeling of my up coming procedure.

Dec. 14, 2015

Pre-indoctrination to the day of my surgery.

My hospital has a great program for people who have pending surgery. This is to have what I would label as a concierge for the hospital. They have a person who's total job is to take you around to the first place you will check in to on your day of surgery, walk you through each of the locations you will be taken, show you your location of surgery, and then the room (or one like it) where you will end up for your two night stay while recovering. I felt this was a great idea in that I

knew exactly where I was going to go to check in,

then the next step, and where I would end up. My wife was along with me so she was aware of the same information. This prevents misunderstandings in time and place situations and makes the entire procedure much more streamlined.

You are going to be thinking about a lot of things on that day and probably be feeling considerable pressure and maybe some uncertainty, you don't need any "Curve balls" being thrown at you. This makes you feel like it's the *second* time you've done this, so you really have a handle on it, and therefore there are very few surprises.

Dec. 22, 2015
Day of surgery

Finally, the day I have been planning on, looking forward to, and the day on which I have been focusing since August. First of all they tell you not to eat or drink anything after 12 am midnight. So no breakfast for me, not even coffee. Sacrifices must be made!

Instructions are to arrive at the hospital, Building 1 at 12:00 pm to check in. I arrive, present my ID card and am check in, then we go to the Ortho Surgery floor and one of the staff greets us and gives me a surgical robe with instructions to put it on and wait in the appointed room. Shortly after that a tech person comes in and instructs me to lie down on this gurney, when I do they start an IV in me to administer fluids. However; the "Sticker" as my wife calls the one sticking you with the needle, cannot hit the correct vein, so he brings in another nurse to do the job. Finally they get me "Hooked up" and off I go to a waiting room until approximately 3:00 pm. Finally it's time! They wheel me into to the surgery room where they only do knee/hip replacements, and explain that they are going to give me a "Spinal Tap" (Nothing to do with the band of that name, although we joke about it), because it has a much faster recovery time that general anesthetic. I am a little bit apprehensive because I thought I was going to be totally zonked out, but they told me that I was going to have a very light "Twilight type" drug administered so I would not be too much aware of the procedure. They were right, it was a little more than what I would consider "Twilight". I don't remember a single thing except a voice saying, "Wake up now, it's time to get you back to your room." The recovery time was much shorter than the standard general anesthetic I could remember from my last knee operation 30 years ago.

Now I am in my private room for the next 2 days, and I actually feel pretty good as far as a low level of pain, and have a good general feeling of well being. I told one of the nurse techs, "Hey this isn't so bad for a pain level, and I thought it would be worse. She says, "You see that tube attached to your arm? It's delivering what is called Morphine, it's got a lot to do with that absence of pain. You won't be taking that with you, so don't get too attached to it!" Little did I know what was coming as it was related to painkillers, but for now I was a happy camper.

Dec. 22, 2015
First night after surgery

My first night there was pretty good minus the fact that the techs and or nurses must come around every hour and check on you, and to do that they have to *wake you up*! Naturally I don't get much sleep, and the next day I would love to sleep, but it daylight, and people are coming and going, no less than 5 or 6 doctors, nurses, techs and other staff are floating in and out of my room with questions about how I feel, do I need to use the bathroom, etc. All of the staff are very professional and personable, and just doing their job that they are assigned. I realize this and do my best to shut up, and use words like "Thanks…I'm doing great, no problems here", and so on.

First Day after surgery
Get on up! Before the end of the day that's what they're telling me. They bring in a walker (which will be MY walker to take home), and the next thing I know it we are going for a stroll down the hallway where I'm actually putting weight on my "New knee", and it all seems pretty natural. I'm thinking, "That Morphine stuff…is that all gone"? I notice there's no more needle in my arm, and my

knee is starting to send me an "Iter-body" text message saying, "Hey…could we get some more if that same stuff we had earlier, because things are starting to get a little hairy with the pain thing down here?"

That's when they introduce the pain killer *pills*. They wanted me to try different pain medications to see how each one reacted to my body. The first one was called "Norco" (Not the town just east of Riverside Ca.) and it didn't have much of an effect on my pain, so they said "Here, try this, it's called *Percocet*." I said, "Now that's what I'm talking about, yeah baby. I'll be taking some of that stuff home with me."

I won't go into it now, but you will want to read the chapter on "Drug dependency" ***long before*** you need a pain killer.

Second night in hospital
Now on the pain killer Percocet, I still feel pretty good, the staff is still coming around on a regular basis to give me blood pressure tests, and of course one of the pills every 4 hours. That is the dosage recommended for the drug. It you're in a lot of pain you can take 2 every 4 hours, but for the way

it made me feel, if I took 2, I would *really* be in "La la Land". If I could describe the feeling I'd say it's *not* something I would want to do for "Fun", it's kind of like you're in this fog of slight numbness, where things can just "Twirl" for an instant, then you're back to what *seems* like reality. Everyone says you've got to be very careful of that stuff, because you can get addicted very easily. Now that's something I can't imagine, because to get addicted, you've got to really like something, right? There is no way I could ever like the feeling of walking around in "Gah gah land" intentionally, wanting to take a knap all the time. But that's just me.

Dec. 24 Christmas Eve Day
Second day after surgery (In hospital)

I wake up feeling pretty good, sun is shining through the window, I get breakfast, and the pain is now a little more noticeable, but still tolerable. My physical therapist tells me today we are going to learn to walk up a flight of stairs. This is good, because that's how I am going to get to my 2nd story bedroom at home. This is employing the use of a cane, and I have the ultimate cane. It's made of bamboo, fire hardened, with a crook on the top and rubber tip on the bottom. People don't know it, but a standard cane with a crook at the top is also a very effective martial arts weapon as used for hundreds of years by the Chinese older monks, and has been carried in the back seat of my truck for 16 years, but more on that later. Today is the day they let me come home.
At about 3:00 pm they notify me that I am going to be released and can go home. They put me in a

wheelchair and take me down to the pick up area, I am actually able to put some weight on the knee and get into the car my wife has waiting for me and we are on our way. I feel like I just broke out of Sing Sing.

Dec. 24, 2015
Christmas Eve at home

My wife made some dinner, and then went over to her Sister's for a family gathering, I didn't feel like going and pressing my luck with my new prosthetic device. I would have to be getting in and out of a car, walking up a driveway and sidewalk, negotiating obstacles, and all that. I took root on the couch with a coffee table in front of me, to prop my leg up, and the TV remote taped to my hand. I was king of my domain and could watch whatever I wanted, but no wine or alcohol. It was kind of a bitter/sweet situation. The Percocet was keeping the pain at a manageable level and I was thinking, "This could be worse". Little did I know it was going to get a lot worse as far as getting off the Percocet, but that is for another chapter.

Dec. 25, 2015

Christmas day

I ventured out of the house for the first time with my brand new walker, and we went over to my

Sister-in-law's for the Christmas dinner and celebration. Actually it was easier that I thought,

and the walker was a real necessity. I was learning to put more weight on the knee, and the Percocet wasn't making me too "Ga ga" to be able to enjoy the day and the people around me. I've never taken a major pain killer, like the Opiates, and didn't know what to expect as far as side effects, and the like. In my case it just felt like I was in a slight fog, and once in a while things would spin for a half of a second, and you're thinking, "Whoa, I'm glad I've got this walker." It really changes your life style and limits your mobility, not to mention, you won't be doing any driving for about a month or more. You may as well face it, your life is not going to be the same for about 6 to 7 weeks.

Dec. 26,2015 – Jan 10, 2016
The next few weeks

Basically I settled into a pattern of doing things, these are things that I was not use to doing, but needed to do to insure success with my new joint replacement. Some of these things were:

Self-injections – Clot prevention
LOVENOX injections: This is a drug self-administered by injection to thin the blood in order to prevent clotting in the leg or any other part of the body. I was sent home with 6 syringe needles to be self-administered each day until all were

gone. You just pinch a flap of skin on your stomach and stick it in, push the plunger and that's that. They have a special type of syringe/needle assembly that once you use it, you push the end plunger, and a protector cap snaps over the end of the needle to prevent accidental puncture of anyone holding or transporting it. Then it is put in a secure area with the other used needles, and dropped off at the hospital's depository for such things the next time you go in.

Compression Socks

As previously mentioned compression socks prevent blood clots in the lower leg and should be worn at night. You can take them off for 2 hours a day to wash them. These can be difficult to on because you will most likely have standard socks on to keep your toes warm, since these socks are not closed at the ends. It is best to put on the compression socks first and then the standard socks. Since you will not be able to bend your leg for the first few weeks you will need help in doing this.

What could go "Wrong"

There are a lot of things that can go "Wrong" with an operation like this, or can develop "Complications" as they say. Infection is the worst enemy you have to worry about, because if one little "Bug" gets in there past the stitches, or you happen to bump your knee or your hip, or worst case scenario succumb to a fall, you are going to be in big trouble. They will have to bring you back in, open you up, find the trouble, fix it, and you start all over again. That's why in the first couple of weeks after coming home it is very critical that you use extra care in everything you do as far as your mobility, and moving around your home.

As mentioned before, remove all throw rugs, unnecessary furniture or obstructions. It's going to be hard enough navigating your pathways around your home using a walker or even a cane, you don't need to make it any harder.

If you have hardwood floors, that is a good thing, it helps in that you won't be catching the outside of your shoe or slipper on the carpet, and doing an imitation of the "I've fallen, and I can't get up" lady.

You will develop an intrinsic ability to become more and more efficient in calculating the items you need around you when you go from one place to another, like from the kitchen to the couch. You'll ask yourself *before* you sit down, "Where are my glasses, is that blanket within reach, is the phone close by, and where IS my cell phone anyway." It seems like once you get settled in your place of "Recline" there's always something you need that's out of reach, and you feel guilty asking some to get it for you.

Month of February - Physical Therapy

Now I am in my 5th week of having my new knee installed and still taking the painkiller Percocet. I have had several physical therapy sessions with a therapist that has come to the house to help me learn the different exercises I must constantly keep doing in order to break up scar tissue, and increase muscular strength, as well as exercising the new joint. She is a very personable lady, good at what she does and I see our sessions as very valuable.

Scar tissue
After the operation this is your biggest issue, breaking up this scar tissue that forms in the area of the joint replacement. It will limit your level of flexibility, and if not dealt with in the first 2 months, you will be permanently limited as to how well you can bend your knee or hip.
After scar tissue forms in the body, it is not permanent. The scar tissue can become stronger

and better able to tolerate stretching forces through a process called remodeling. Remodeling scar tissue is a must to ensure that the muscle, tendon, skin, bone, or ligament becomes normal, healthy tissue again. This restructuring or remodeling process is painful. Scar tissue remodeling occurs as you start to stretch and pull on it. The stretching of the scar tissue helps to align the collagen fibers to allow them to return to normal. This realignment of the collagen fibers makes the tissue better able to tolerate the forces that are placed on it during the day. You need to stretch the lower leg in both directions (leg flat and leg bent), and that will be painful.

Leg flat

This is accomplished by laying your leg flat on a soft surface and pushing against that surface (or having someone else push on your knee cap downward) so that your leg is as flat or even has a negative angle against the surface. A good way to help this exercise along in a passive manner is to sit on a couch or chair, put the heel of your foot on another support (like a coffee table) and just rest it there as long as you can, letting the weight of your leg bend it in a negative angle. If you really want to help it along you can put a light weight (like a book or full water bottle) on it for a short while.

Leg bent

Next you need to achieve the most acute angle between your lower leg and your thigh. For some people this is more difficult, and causes the most pain in breaking up that scar tissue. You can sit lengthwise on a couch with the arm as a back rest, and draw your ankle up toward your thigh by putting a belt around your ankle, and pulling your ankle up as close to your thigh as the pain will allow. Hold to 10 seconds and relax. Over the weeks each time you repeat it, you will get better at achieving a greater and sharper angle between your calf and your upper leg.

Now I am going in to the actual physical therapy location at Kaiser, and working with a professional therapist.

My physical therapist would measure this angle with a plastic protractor that would get a very accurate measurement. My goal for flexibility was 140 degrees. This was very difficult for me to get to this point, so he said, “Here, let me help you”, later on, I learned every time he said that, it involved me experiencing a considerable amount of pain! So, he just with very exacting pressure forced my lower leg up toward my thigh. I soon found out what real pain was (and I was on the painkillers). Once again he said, “You can hate me now (for doing my job) or hate me later for taking it easy on you.” Meaning if he didn’t help

me really break up the scar tissue, then I would not have the flexibility later, forever. I think of this every time I bend my leg back.

Gym workouts

At some point you are going to have to take on the responsibility for doing your own therapy, in between your professional therapy visits. You are going to need access to some professional gym machines to do the necessary exercises to get your leg muscles back into shape.

ATROPHY: The wasting away of muscular parts because of non-use or damage. This is what happens to your thigh and calf muscles because you have not used them for 2 months. Although you need to exercise the new joint, you also need to get back your muscular strength that you've lost by not using your leg or putting any stress on it for at least 4 weeks. If you have joined or belong to a gym where they have the machines necessary to provide the exercises like the stationary bike, the leg press machine, and the kick exerciser, then you are in good shape…if you use it.

The trouble with a lot of people is, they don't have the motivation to get off the couch, quit watching daytime TV, and go use your membership.

Chapter 5
Observations & tips

Drug Rehab – The worst part of the experience

You've always heard somebody say", Now don't get addicted to that "Thing you're doing".

You are going to be taking a pain killer pill that is very strong, and effects different people different ways and levels. In killing pain, this drug also has some side effects that some people might like. A feeling of euphoria, and floating, along with weightlessness.

Bottom line: You may start to like this stuff, but when you do , you won't know you like this stuff, until it's too late.
So…don't getting to like this too much, because you can't have this all the time, and still have a life!

In my case I was taking only 1 – 3.5 mg every four hours, that was the dosage in the prescription. I did this for 6 weeks. I used the 4 hr. mark as evaluation of how much pain I was feeling in knee, and your hip is much the same thing. As the 4 hour mark came up I began to feel the pain become more acute and I was "Ready" for another pill. I didn't have to worry about waking up in the night or early am to take one, my knee woke me up.

Pill intake tip:
Cut a piece of paper the size of the pill bottle and wrap it around the outside, and secure it with clear scotch tape. Then write the time you should take a pill within the next 24 hour period down the side. Ex: If taking one every 4 hours write 8 – 12 – 4 – 8 – 12am down the side. When you take one, put a check mark by that number. There will come a time when after you take a pill, or should take one, that you will think, “Did I just take a pill or not?” You don’t want to double up on intake, and you certainly don’t want to forget to take one. This will eliminate any indecision.

As far as “Liking” the drug Percocet, I would never like to have that in my system unless it was for major pain. I am too much of a “Gotta have control” type of person, and don’t like surrendering my brain, and body to a drug. Knowing this, you’ve got to realize that your body gets “accustomed” to the physical need of some substances, and even though your mental state says “I don’t need this stuff”, your body is saying, “Wait a minute, I kind’a like this stuff”. It’s called physical dependency, and it doesn’t take long for it to happen. It is almost a given fact that you are going to be in a fluctuating degree of dependency to this (or what ever drug you have chosen) substance for help with your pain, even when you don’t need it to help with your pain. That is when you have got another problem to deal with.

Getting "Off" the pain killer

Now we are talking about one of the most important aspects of your entire experience of your operation. When you get the pills from your pharmacy they attach a folded piece of paper that when unfolded looks almost a big as a sail for a catamaran. In this dissertation of "Cover your own ass" statements that every drug company has seen fit to issue, are warnings, and projections of do's
and don'ts, as well as the typical withdrawal symptoms you can experience when getting of this drug. I however, neglected to read the part that said, "*After prolonged use, do not quit taking Percocet with out a prolonged program of gradual reduced intake.*" In other words don't quit "Cold turkey". It goes on to describe the withdrawal symptoms if you choose to do this.
In the 5 week of my taking the drug, I felt that the pain in my knee was significantly reduced and I didn't need to take a pain killer any more, so I did quit, cold turkey. Once again, I should have read that disclaimer!

It wasn't long before I experienced cold sweats, and overheating, the inability to sleep, and a strange feeling that someone was tickling the inside of my chest with a feather, that just got worse unless I got up and walked around. It was like a little ball of energy was forming in my chest or stomach and was getting bigger and more pronounced. I would have to get up and shake myself or expend energy or it felt like I would explode. Then in a few minutes I would have to do it again.

I had to go to the drug dependency clinic in my health plan to get counseling and help with this problem. It was at least 3 weeks before this symptom would dissipate, and I still have bouts of the anxiety at night, and eventually it took 50 days before I could get back to my life as I knew it before taking the drug.

I went on line and searched the term *Percocet withdrawal symptoms*, and read the posts from people that were taking the drug because of chronic pain or longer lasting problems, more than just a knee or hip replacement. Now reading their stories made me feel like I had no problems at all, because a lot of these people were in very bad shape with all kinds of pain related issues.

I have been told that specifically Percocet stays in your system for a total of over one month. It was my experience that even past that time of quitting the drug I could not even have a glass of wine in the evening or I would be up with the same withdrawal symptoms all night. Finally when I got to the 50th day after taking the drug, I could have a glass of champagne or wine without experiencing the wakeup at 2:00 am with the withdrawal symptoms of anxiety and sleeplessness. I was also told by my therapist that alcohol magnifies the latent effects of pain killers, if there is any amount remaining in your system. As previously mentioned, each person is different in their reaction to pain and drugs. How it affects you is personal and you should recognize these effects as quickly as possible, but a good policy is, "Less is better", and of course always check with your doctor immediately when encountering any problems.

PAIN

Pain is a very strange phenomenon, in that if effects different people in different ways, and everyone has a different level of pain tolerance, and ways of handling it.

One of the related feelings pain inflicted on me was the hyper-sensitivity of cold and warm temperatures. If it was one or two degrees difference I would feel like I was freezing or roasting. I would get overheated very easily, and then in a few minutes I would be shivering. It was constantly, "Honey, would you turn that heat up, I'm freezing here", or "Turn that dog gone heat off will 'ya, I'm roasting here"! Thank goodness my wife and caretaker for 2 mo., is a very tolerant and wonderful person.

STRANGE PAIN

Another strange pain I encountered was a sudden jolt, which felt like an electric shock just went through my knee and up my leg. I wasn't even moving, just had my foot up on the couch, my knee was in a bent position, totally immobile, no pressure on it in any way, and WHAM! This bolt of lightning zaps me like I was hooked up to 110 volts from the wall outlet. Someone told me it was possibly a nerve trying to reconnect. This happened no less that 15 or 20 times and still happens once in a while.

Bottom line about drug withdraws is, don't wait to get help if you feel you have a problem getting off of whatever you are taking, because the chances of you getting better by yourself are slim. There's usually only one direction for withdrawal and it's down hill, so don't wait until you think it's just going to get better by itself, the chances are not in your favor. Most people do need help, JUST DO IT!"

CONSTIPATION

Oh yes…this is one problem pain killers will inflict upon you. I didn't "Go" for 5 days, even while taking laxatives. When I did it was not pleasant, and it looked like someone threw a 6' black bullwhip in the toilet!

This creates a catch 22 problem, especially for older people who may have heart problems or anomalies. There is a phenomena called the Valsalva's maneuver in which a person is straining to have a bowel movement and this act puts undue pressure on the heart, and can cause a heart attack. So, you are in need of getting rid of this waste in your body, you're bound up, but you shouldn't strain because you don't want to make it tough on your heart. What do you do?

Suppositories are one avenue to try, and of course you should be taking some form of laxative. A cup of coffee has always solved that problem for me, so much in that I can't even think of having a cup if I am going to drive any distance on the freeway. How you solve the problem is up to you, but the word here is, "Forewarned is forearmed" and best of luck.

ALCOHOL

For the people who would like to have their favorite alcoholic related beverage while recovering, don't even *think* about it. In that previously mentioned large piece of paper containing all the disclaimers, and instructions about the drug you are taking, it tells you in no uncertain terms that alcohol and drugs (of any kind) do not mix. In addition, you most likely have been give a healthy dose of some kind of antibiotic or are taking one now to prevent infection. This further pushes the risk of bad things happening if you "Fall off the wagon" of sobriety. It comes under the umbrella of "Sacrifices must be made", and this is one you really don't want to toy with.

To help you with this longing, take a glass and put some soda pop, sparkling water, or your favorite juice in it along with a few ice cubes. It will give you much of the same sensation that

you *are* having a "Drink", without the ramifications. Sometimes you just want something to drink while working or watching TV, and this seems to fill the bill.

DIETARY SUPPLEMENTS

Before the operation I was taking glucosamine sulfate, fish oil, aspirin, (aspirin was suspended a week before the operation to keep from thinning my blood) and for cholesterol, Atorvastatin, and for my heart Atrial Fibrillation, Metoprolol to slow down my heart beat. I was told to resume taking these drugs a week after I returned home.

One of the things to consider after an operation like this is the fact that you have lost a considerable amount of blood. My doctor mentioned this, and the fact that I could become anemic and have iron deficiency. I was feeling a little weak at times, and when I had the blood work done after the operation the results supported that assumption, so I was told to take iron pills, one a day, for 30 days to help correct this deficiency. Iron does tend to make your stool very dark or black, so don't freak out. Before taking any supplements it is highly recommended to get the blood work done if you haven't already, to be sure you are on the right track. Of course you should consult your doctor before taking any supplements, or drugs of any kind, and of course read all the disclaimers posted in the drug instructions given when you receive the tablets.

Chapter 6
Physical Rehabilitation

You have gone through a lot by now, and will end up paying a healthy amount of money as a co-pay for this operation. It would be a major waste of everything expended if you were not to recover the maximum degree of flexibility and movement you could attain by the implementation of the proper physical therapy. Some health plans provide payment of therapy, some you have to provide yourself. Which ever one you have, it is of major importance that you either have a professional physical therapist to guide you through the necessary steps, and
exercises to regain as much flexibility and range of motion that you had long before you needed this replacement.

Professional help

As previously mentioned in the words of my physical therapist, as he was forcing my lower leg up toward my upper leg to break up some of the scar tissue, “You can hate me now or hate me later” (for the rest of your life). You only have about 2 months to break up this scar tissue that will form around your knee, and keep you from bending it at the maximum angle that would give you the most flexibility. Beyond that, there is no going back. So most doctors and patients who've done this, say that you really need to hire a professional physical therapist. They will keep you on the right pathway, and make sure you are doing the exercises correctly, with the right amount of weight, and repetitions. Most medical facilities have within them a physical therapy department. If they don't, they most likely can recommend a certified therapist that will fill the bill. The bottom line is, JUST DO IT!

Getting your life back

In the second month of your adventure in becoming partially a "Bionic" human being, you have settled into getting use to being on a pain killer that prevents you from doing a lot of things you would like to do as well as things you would *have* to do if it were not for this "Detour" you've taken in life.

You have gotten use to limited mobility, having to get use to using a walker, then a cane, and now maybe limping around your environment to get what you need from parts of your house etc.
As the weeks go by you are meeting these challenges and settling in to believe that's the way things are going to be for a while.

LIFE DISRUPTIONS

For the next 45 days your life will not be the same, you will go through many changes that will be physical as well as mental. Some people handle change better that others, how you react to these changes and disruptions it up to you. Keep in mind that in 2 to 3 months you will be back in action, and your life will be better, more pain free, and more mobile that ever before. Remember: *"Nothing is as difficult or as easy as it appears, the second time you look at it".* So, whatever your perception of the situation you are in, step back and take that second look. It's going to get better.

For me the major life disruptions were:

No driving - (on painkillers) This is a major subtraction of a very needed self-service. It means you cannot go to the grocery store or any retail outlet. You must get someone else to drive you. Which makes you dependent on someone else for this, so you are "House bound" for at least 30 - 45 days, or until you get off the painkillers.

No showers, Jacuzzi or pool action: Until the stitches heal totally you cannot get the area wet. This means you have to take "Sponge baths", and since I love a Jacuzzi to help my joints all over, this was a major set back, at least for 20 or more days.

Reduced awareness – The painkiller you're taking tends to make you less aware of your surroundings, the ability to make decisions, follow a plan of action, even choose words and phrases that make sense. I found myself trying to recall the name of a prominent actor…blank. Walked into to the kitchen to get ice…blank out. Trying to use my computer, I forgot which program I was in. This can be scary, but it doesn't last forever. Hang in there, it will get better.

Time allotment shift – Let's examine your day as far as how your time was metered out for what you accomplished. This is a description of my day the way it use to be.

BEFORE THE OPERATION.

8 am – 9 am: Get up, make breakfast, eat breakfast, watch news, and arrange data for contacting potential healthcare clients.
9 am – 11:30 – Talk to clients and potential clients interested in becoming part of my healthcare program and work on web site changes etc.
12:00 pm – 3:00 pm Teaching and or playing tennis in the local area.
3:00 pm – 4:30 pm – Soaking in the Jacuzzi, swimming laps in the pool.
4:30 pm – 6:00 pm – Working on one of my books or magazine articles

6:00 – Bedtime – Relaxing, watching news, reading etc.
The previous time map of my day was approximately 9 to 10 hours of constant activity before my operation.

AFTER THE OPERATION

Take that 10 hours of activity and wipe it off the map! From the time I got home until 45 days later my major activity was switching TV channels from the Tennis Channel, to the Andy Griffith show, punctuated by knap time for an hour or more. The biggest deviation was icing my knee with the cold water machine, on and off every half hour. I'm not going to be driving, going in the Jacuzzi, and definitely not teaching or playing any tennis, so for an active person like me, it wasn't easy. Take 8 or more hours of constant activity and reduce it to zero activity.

Because I was on the painkillers for much of that time, I really could not talk to clients or potential clients in relation to selling my healthcare program, and it was difficult to answer incoming calls in regards to my self-improvement web site, so all things considered, I was pretty much useless to my revenue producing behavior.

When you consider what you do on a day to day basis including all the activities, and how they take up your day, in makes for a faster pace, and lifestyle. Now you take that same person, and realize they can do none of those things. They are also incapacitated somewhat because of the drugs and pain, can't sleep at night, and you have a maniac without a straightjacket.

Not being able to drive a car, go into a Jacuzzi, and of course enjoy my sport of tennis with friends. This was the longest 2 months of my existence, and the time just dragged on, not to mention the sleepless nights, and drug with drawl symptoms.

I thank my lucky stars, and God, for giving me the most wonderful woman in the world to help me through this, my wife Susan. She was just awesome in making this always painful (even with the Percocet) and stressful time bearable for me. I'm just a lucky guy, and I know it.

Getting it together

Now at the end of the second month, you have permission to step up your workouts at the gym, you can walk without a limp, and are feeling pretty good. As the weeks go buy, you've done a lot of work, gone to the gym, rode the bike, use the leg resistance machine, and are doing all the prescribed exercises. How long is the time period before you can get back did doing the sport You really enjoy, or just a normal lifestyle?

That is a very difficult expansive of time to calculate. For each person there is a different time value. I was told as far as getting back on the tennis court I was to wait three months.

At the end of the Second month I decided to go out and hit a few serves on the tennis court, and I was surprised at my lack of performance and ability. You just don't realize how weak your body can get with the lack of continued use.

As I begin to hit balls I realized that my shoulder was not even close to the capabilities I once had. That should have come as no big realization because I had not hit a ball for eight weeks. Now suddenly I am expecting my shoulder and arm to do the same job as it did when it was in shape. It doesn't take long for your body to get out of shape, and weak when you don't use it for a couple of months.

I had to hit about 60 balls before I was able to get one over the net. I am glad I did not go out and actually try to play in a real game situation.

Someone once said, "Sometimes your mind writes a check that your body just cannot cash." That day I was writing a lot of bad checks, and I realized I had a lot of physical therapy to do on my upper body as well as my knee. The problem with changing and developing your body is, it doesn't happen overnight. It takes time, and that's usually the reason people don't workout, and do the exercises, they don't get immediate gratification or don't see the results soon enough. Whatever sport you enjoy, or physical activity you like to throw yourself into, there is one thought you should keep in mind.

TAKE IT SLOW!

That part of your knee, leg or hip, needs to grow around the prosthetic that was installed in you, and you need to give it a fighting chance. It needs exercise, but controlled exercise, not
abrupt jolting or pressure.

So do the prescribed exercises you were given, and the repetitions prescribed, and as the pain goes away, and the joint swelling goes down, you can ad more weight, and repetitions etc.

If you are an active person wanting to get back to your favorite sport, and an active life, you must guard against putting too much pressure on this new prosthetic device that your body is trying to get use to. You are at the crossroads of your re-development to get back to being better than you were before the operation. One wrong turn in your actions of development like pressing your joint too much, involving yourself in a game related situation where your automatic reactions would put too much pressure on the new joint, and you could set yourself back to before the operation.

It is not worth it, once again take it slow, it's better to go slower than you need to, rather than the other direction, and do damage to your new joint.

It cannot be said too many times: When in doubt of what to do always consult your surgeon or primary care doctor.
Once again: *Life is not a video tape, there is no rewind, no replay!*

My first time on the tennis court

This was a great experience because for the first time in 7 years I could actually take a couple of quick steps putting weight on my right leg without pain. I was able to move (with reasonable care) to the ball getting into position. It was not like I could run or sprint, and then stop suddenly, that may come some day in the distant future, but for now I am just thankful to be back on the court even in a limited capacity. As previously mentioned, I was severely out of shape as far as my upper body strength, and endurance. This is something that I began to work on with regularity, and now 3 and a half months later am just beginning to get back to the place I was 6 months ago before the operation, but I've got a ways to go.

Controlled Stress

In getting back to my "Original self", I noticed the next day after I went out on the tennis court and just hit a few serves, or rallied with someone, my knee would be giving me that signal, "You shouldn't have done that." So I would lay off putting any "Spontaneous" stress on it. That's the dangerous part of going back to your sport that you love so much, because after years of instant reaction to the sports situational challenge (fast reaction to a incoming ball, or charging competitor) you just react, BANG, and you don't think about how much stress you put on your joint or how quick you have to be, it's just automatic. There's no "Half-try" or holding back, because it's once again…AUTOMATIC! That's the kind of stuff you want to stay away from until your 3 months of rehab have gone by, or longer. That bone has got to grow around that post they drove into your lower leg and grow around it to a good degree. If it was a hip replacement, your hip area needs to do the same thing. If you keep over stressing the joint, even if it feels what you think to "OK", it can set you back in your healing.

Your exercise needs to be more controlled in that you want to stress the muscles, without over stressing the prosthetic device against the bone, which is trying to grow around it.

Getting in "Shape"

Our bodies were made to be used, stressed, and pushed to limits we thought were beyond our capabilities. It is only when you do this that your body begins to respond with the powers that it's capable of, many times greater that you give yourself credit for, and it will surprise you.

Getting my body back in shape I found was a slow process, and since I'm such an "Immediate gratification" kind of person I had to push myself to go to the gym and do the workouts to regain the strength I once had. I had to push and motivate myself to do it because it wasn't any "Fun", and the results are not instantly apparent. Riding the stationary bike, using the resistance machines, and or weights is not high on a person's list of fun things to do.

I happen to have adopted a sport that causes a person to burn a lot of calories, while competing, and having that "Fun" previously mentioned. Each time you play there is only one winner and one loser, (2 in doubles). You feel great when you win, and if you don't you analyze why you didn't, but the bottom line is, you enjoy playing the game and you burned an extreme amount of calories in the process. Another aspect of any athletic competition is that the outcome is totally unpredictable, providing that all competitors are in the same ballpark of proficiency. So when people enter in to this arena of competition they both do so with the attitude that *they* will be the winner. This attitude is what makes things interesting, and keeps your interest in the sport, trying to increase your level of proficiency, and constantly be a better player.

On the other hand if you're a person who does not enjoy a "Calorie burning" sport that is fun to do, you have to find a way to burn those calories, put stress on your body in a way to let it know it's being "Used", because you know the old saying, "Use it or lose it."

Learn something new

Some people feel like they are not suited to skill sports, because they are not "Naturally" athletic. They were never encouraged to play sports when they were young, never had brothers or sisters that they could enjoy even the easiest of skill sports like pitch and catch, basketball, baseball etc. It is this kind of person that will find it difficult to bounce back from an operation that leaves them immobile for a period of time, and therefore causes them to become even more out of shape that usual. If you're this kind of person you should take the suggestion to heart that you need to learn a new calorie burning sport. The "Learning" part will help exercise your mind as well as developing your body, and intern boost the adrenaline and endorphin levels in your body, getting the "Juices" flowing. This increases circulation and can increase your general level of energy. As always, make sure to consult your doctor before starting any program of exercise, or taking up a new sport, to see if you are healthy enough to do so. Once again, adopt the idea that whatever you do, you start out slowly, and work in to it. If it is a skill sport like tennis or golf, realize that these are two of the most "Easiest looking – hardest doing", sports you can pick, so get a good instructor, and don't get discouraged. The best part about learning a sport is the mental as well as physical changes you will go through in doing so. You may want to start with a sport that takes less skill, like bike ridding. It will get your heart rate up, develop your legs and cardiovascular areas, and take you places you've never been at a slower pace than just driving. Once again remember the action mantra…JUST DO IT!

Chapter 7
NEW ADDITION TO THIS PRINTING
(The "Other" knee replaced)
The same, but different

The 2nd Time Around - What's different, what's the same.

If you've ever done something or been part of a project that was successful and you find yourself needing to re-create that same project or event over again with the same or better results, what to do you do?

If you're like most people, you try to remember all of the positive things about the event or project, because you'd like to use them again and hopefully get the same results. The trouble with that is, unless you've kept fairly good records, receipts, and notes to jog your memory, there are usually several different pieces of information that somehow get left out or fall through the cracks of time and space we call "Limbo", and when we are re-introduced to those forgotten facts or memories we think, "Oh ya, now I remember why that didn't go the way I'd planned before", and for the same reason this event is going down the same path AS before, and you think, "I've got to keep better notes!"

Bottom line, in my case, (because I have two knees) when you decide to have that same procedure done, or embark on the same type of adventure, or project, *again*, at several points in the project you realize there were things you totally forgot and you have to re-learn them all over.

I now realize why a woman will have more the one child. She forgets all the pain, frustration, and life changing developments she went through the first time. Maybe it's the pain, the bodily changes, and all the rest of the complicated stuff associated with childbirth. At the time, most women have been known to say, "Well I'm never going to do that again"! Yet they do.

As you have previously read, I got my first knee replacement in 2016, and it was all new, I had very little advance knowledge on what to expect, how I was going to react to all of the new stimuli and so because it was all new, it was kind of fun learning experience, even the bad stuff, like the withdrawal symptoms of the Percocet pain killer, and wearing of the compression socks, constant pain for the first 2 weeks, even with the pain killers. It was all new experiences. And, at the end I did say, "Well, I'm *never* doing that again."

Fast forward 2 1/2 years and I am experiencing the same pain and difficulties with my left knee as the right one that was replaced. At least I had a year of playing tennis like I was 40 years old again, so now it's time to have the other knee "Fixed". In deciding to have the procedure again, I thought, "Oh ya, let's do it, it wasn't really that tough of a thing to go through, and it was very successful. WRONG! There was a lot of things that I forgot about that were not the best memories in the world, and that's why I'm adding this last chapter to let people know how I viewed the same procedure, the same experiences etc. but not ***exactly.***

Some of the things that were different:

PAIN: With this type of major surgery there would be a significant amount of pain, if you didn't have some type of painkiller. Since every type of pain killer works different for different people, the hospital will try different types on you to see which is best, with the least amount of putting your physical and mental state in "Gogga land". The first one I was given was called, Norco, and I found out it did basically nothing to help the pain, so they said "Here try this, it's called Percocet."

I thought, "*Now this is what I'm talk'in about!* It was more successful at knocking the pain, but also successful in knocking me out too. I guess that's why people get hooked on it. Back in 2016 nobody was writing articles about it, how hundreds of people were using it "Recreationally", there were no headlines in the newspapers or specials on TV about people OD-ing on it when combined with other drugs etc. Personally I can't stand the feeling of being in "La La Land" but if it was necessary to keep the pain at bay…so be it.

The noticeable difference between this recent new knee installation and the first one, was that the surgeons put a nerve blocker (injected) in the knee area of the leg in question. Which is just like shooting all the pain medicine into the one spot where it's needed. I got home and felt that this whole pain thing was just somebody's way of wimping out and complaining. WRONG! I told my wife about how great I felt and she said, "*Before you start moonwalking across the living room, remember that nerve blocker they shot you up with? It's not going to last forever.*" Whoa, was she right! The next morning, I couldn't wait to slap that ice pack on, and spend the day watching the golf channel (when I was awake).

Now I'm experiencing what is called bearable pain, but…the new drug they added to my painkillers was a Morphine pill, to be taken every 8 hours. That seemed to do the trick to managing the pain, but I was just a little "Ga Ga", not totally out of it, but on the edge. Everything was a little foggy, and I always wanted to take a knap all the time.

WITHDRAWALS: In remembering the bad withdrawal symptoms of the last time with Percocet I was wondering what this would be like.

Since you've already read the previous information about the negative effect of quitting Percocet cold turkey (It tells you NOT to do that in the instructional pamphlet you get with the drugs) you may be wondering how the Morphine tablet was going to work along side the Percocet. I found it to be very effective, and did a lot to bring the pain level down to a manageable level with just one Percocet of 500 mg, last time I was taking 2.

A this writing I am just getting off of the Percocet, or at least tapering off to only 1/2 tablet per 8 hours and then only 1/4 as the last intake just before sleep at 11 pm. Well I guess my body didn't like the total amount it was getting because that night was filled with the same kind of explosive high energy that caused me to have to sit up in bed, move around, breathe deeply and try to get to sleep. The trouble is, the minute you close your eyes the same thing starts happening all over again. It's crazy, it feels like you've had 5 cups of coffee, on the night before you've got to give a business presentation that will either make or break your company, and you've lost all your notes. Your mind is flying with unrelated thoughts, and you want to just get up and read a book, have some warm milk, or a sleeping pill. Anyway, I must have broke through this wall of dependency, because I finally got to sleep around 4 am.
They say to drink a lot of water, like force feed yourself water, and to taper off slowly, I guess my body had a altogether different definition of what

“Slowly” was, because I've been off of it now for 8 days and still can't get to sleep for more than a hour at a time. One of the things that made the pain more bearable was the "Cold water" ice machine. Thanks to my wonderful wife, she knew how to keep the machine on me for the right amount of time, when to take it off, and kept a good supply of frozen water bottles in the freezer. As I mentioned in previous text, it's so much easier than using actual ice to produce the cold water, and of course cheaper than buying ice all the time.

So now I'm in my 5th week of convalescence, still have yet to make it through a night without awaking to an "Overcharged" system of high energy. That Percocet is some wild stuff that stays in your system longer that it's suppose to…I think. But that's just me, and everyone has a different reaction to it. When I looked up the different withdrawal symptoms, it sounded like someone was reading a disclaimer for one of the "As seen on TV" drugs. Here are some of the wildly known symptoms: Agitation, Diarrhea, Nausea, Muscle Aches Mood Swings, Insomnia, Sweating, Chills, and Headaches. When you are trying to detox something like this they tell you to drink a lot of water, and that is one thing that helped me. You've just got to remember to drink it, and drink it, and yes…drink it. It's hard to drink water when you don't actually need it because you're thirsty, but do it anyway, it works. You WILL get over this.

▪

Chapter 8
What your day & night will really be like

Ok, so here it is, the "Tell it like is it" part of this book, the unsugar coated depiction of what you are going to experience after coming home. This is the part of the story that will probably be making you realize that this is going to be no picnic, and maybe you want to re-evaluate your decision to do, or not to do this procedure.

First of all my hospital, Kaiser Permanente, which I think did a great job, and is absoutly the best…is now sending people home on the same day as the operation. Good idea if you're in good health, came through it fine and don't really need to spend the night in the hospital or spend the extra money to stay there. It naturally will reduce your bill if you choose to get out of there asap. A night in the hospital is not free.

What your day will be like. Naturally everyone wants to know about the pain, and how much discomfort you may be in. The first day is not so bad because you've got a lot of that painkiller called Morphine, in you. In my case they put a nerve blocker in my leg, which is an injection that does just that, block the nerves responsible for delivering the pain message to your brain. You feel great, and begin to think, "Hey this is gonna be a breeze." Wait awhile Bunkie, it will change. Your best friend will be the walker that was included in the deal with the hospital. Everywhere you go, it will be using the walker, so if you don't have someone to be looking after you 24/7 you'd better get someone, or you're going to be very frustrated after the 4th time you have to get up off whatever couch, bed or Lazyboy, you happen to be making as your at rest home place, just to get a drink, book, or any one of umpteen things you'll want to have near you.

The Ice Machine

This is you second best friend, because it is going to keep the swelling down as much as possible while the knee (or hip) is healing.

It is a one-gallon plastic bucket with a electric pump that supplies ice cold water to a special bladder with many little water pockets designed to transfer that level of cold temperature to your knee. It's a real job to get to rest on your knee in just the right spot, with the elastic bands that have Velcro ends that catch on anything and everything you don't want it to catch on. Your leg must be elevated even with your body so that means that you have to be in a prone position like in bed. But who wants to be in bed all day long so I gravitated over the couch, got a couple of pillows on the coffee table, put my leg up there and kick back with the TV remote in my hand. I've got the tennis and the golf channel at my disposal and life is good!

Compression Socks

Now here's something you might not have been planning on. They usually put these things on you at the end of the operation, but their purpose is to compress the calves of your both legs to improve circulation and prevent blood clots. They are knee length and they are somewhat difficult to get on unless you have a helper, and not a lot of fun to wear. You need to wear them for 5 to 7 weeks. They look great if you're wearing a Scottish kilt on St. Patty's Day, otherwise if you don't like the look, don't wear shorts.

You get to take them off for about 20 minutes a day, so, until you begin to have the ability to bend your knee to an angle that will afford you the ability to get the sock over your toes, this is a task you're going to need help with. It will be just another little diversion in some several parts of your day.

Bathing
For the first couple of weeks you don't want to even think about getting your incision wet, so you are going to be pretty good at what we call "Sponge bathing", once again, it's really helpful if you have someone to help you in that area.

Knapping
Because of the painkillers you are taking, you're very likely to become more than a little drowsy, and get to enjoy a mid-day knap. Depending the time you spend day sleeping will have a very noticeable effect on how well you sleep at night. There is a good chance with most people who do this, their biological clock will begin to change and suddenly you are changing into a rock star, or Weir wolf, sleeping all day and raging all night. Unless you have a mate or

house full of people who enjoy keeping you company at 3:00 am, try to resist the temptation to drop out during the day.

Physical Therapy

THIS is the most important part of your day. You have scar tissue around your knee and it needs to be broken up by flexing the knee to the farthest angle of bend and straightness that you can manage. There are exercises you were given by your doctor, or hospital. Do these exercises without fail! This is not an option! You only have a limited amount of time to regain your flexibility which is about 2 to 3 months and after that what ever level of flexibility you have achieved is all you're going to get. Have a particular time of your day to do these exercises and put as much effort into them as possible. Otherwise you are just wasting all of the time, trouble, and money spent to give you a new joint that will work perfectly, and you won't end up any better that before the replacement. JUST DO IT!

Chapter 9
Interviews and first hand experiences

These are actual real-time interviews with people who have had knee and hip replacements. They were recorded and transcribed exactly as told in audio recordings and face-to-face interviews.

John Doby– Laguna Niguel, Ca.
Age 72
Activities: Tennis player, baseball player, runner
Surgery: Knee replacement & multiple surgeries
Knee surgeries – 1972 -1975 – 1979
Total Knee Replacement – 2013

Q: You had your most recent knee replacement done because of what reason?
A: Could not walk any more, had a lot of pain all the time, and was told it was the only alternative. I wanted to remain active, and at that stage of the game it wasn't possible.

Q: Were there any complications, how did it go?
A: Complications would be an understatement.
I had an issue of blood clots in my leg, a hematoma in the leg where the knee was replaced. The blood clot got to my lung, a pulmonary embolism. I had to have a filter installed to keep the blood clots from getting to my lower body from my upper body. I later developed Polymyalgia Rheumatica.

Definition: Polymyalgia rheumatica is an inflammatory disorder that causes muscle pain and stiffness, especially in the shoulders. Symptoms of polymyalgia rheumatica (pol-e-my-AL-juh rue-MAT-ih kuh) usually begin quickly and are worse in the morning. Most people who develop polymyalgia rheumatica are older than 65. It rarely affects people under 50. Now the rheumatologist said it might be rheumatic arthritis.

Q: So now that the knee is replaced 3 years later, how do you feel, and how is it working?
A: The knee that was replaced is actually quite good, Sometimes I actually walk around 10 miles plus or minus. I was told not to run any more, but I was told that with the first knee operation. I was an avid runner for a lot of years, but now have had to eliminate that from my workouts. But the bottom line my right knee (replaced) is quite good now. My left knee is kind of a problem, but it gets cortisone shots every 3 to for months, and that seems to handle the problem.

Q: So that's the knee you didn't have replaced?
A: Well, I had 2 surgeries done on that knee. It was a medial ligament they had to remove, and cartridge damage in that knee that has not been replaced.

Q: What kind of pain meds did they give you?
A: The prescription they gave me was for Hydrocodone. I took that as needed, it was pretty successful, I didn't take it every 4 hours as it was prescribed.

Q: How difficult was it to wean yourself from the drug?
A: It was pretty seamless, I had no withdrawal symptoms to speak of.

Q: So now you're doing pretty good, sometimes you may have a problem with the other knee once in a while but over all it's all positive.
A: Well, I still have a problem with the RA (Rheumatic arthritis) and now I'm taking Methotrexate for that. RA is carried in your blood and attacks soft joints. 4 or 5 months after the knee replacement surgery I'd wake up after 2 hours of sleep with severe pain in one shoulder and then the other shoulder would be in pain 20 minutes later, so my sleep was increasingly reduced until I was unable to sleep only 15 minutes before the pain would come back. To dissipate the pain I would get up and move around, that would help for a few minutes then the pain would come back. So they treated that with Prednisone, and I am still taking it. That was helpful for about 6 months, now they think it was not the Polymyalgia rheumatic but Rheumatic Arthritis, so they have prescribed the Methotrexate for that, which is an ugly drug, it's almost a Chemotherapy type treatment, so they

give me other drugs to try and reduce the loss of hair, but I'm not sure it's working.

Q: Do you have trouble sleeping now?
A: The Methotrexate seems to be getting it back under control. They increased the dosage, and now it's better and now I'm able to sleep 4 hours at a time.

Byron Nelson – Laguna Ca.
Age: 72
Retired Attorney – Ex College football player & now tennis player, golfer, skier, volleyball player.
2 Knee replacements 2 shoulder replacements

Q: So Byron, what prompted you to get the first knee replacement?
A: Total pain, usability, one I lived with for 30 years, the first one, my knee had totally detrained. The other one happened rapidly, the second one, I slipped and probably tore an ACL in my right knee, so I had to have it done about 6 months later. The second one, I had to have done was 25 years later.

Q: Was it the same hospital?
A: Yes, the same doctor, same hospital. It was 2000 when I had the first one replaced and 2005 when I had the second one replaced.

Q: How long were you in the hospital?
A: The first one I was in the hospital for 3 days, basically incapacitated for that time. The second one was also 3 days, but things have changed drastically so much since then.

Q: When you did come home, how long did it take you to be able to get back into your life again as far as your regular routine and activities?

A: The first one, well things weren't advanced as they are now, and we didn't know quite as much about it all as we do now, but I was using a crutches and limping around right away. I never used a walker. It was about two weeks before I started all the rehab stuff.

Q: How long was it before you could get back on the tennis court and be at least hitting some balls to ease yourself back into the sport?
A: Well I really took it sooner that they told me to, but I waited 3 months before I started to put any pressure on the knee. But, by the 4th month I was doing pretty good.

Q: How long have you been playing tennis?
A Oh, I'd say at least 40 years.

Q: What did you take for painkiller drugs?
A: I didn't take any at all. I've have had 4 joint replacements, and I've never had any pain, except just the first day afterward. I never took any after I left the hospital, never needed it, it's not that I'm that tough, I just didn't experience any pain to speak of. The doctors that did it were excellent, and the results were excellent.

Q: So what other sports do you play?
A: I enjoy skiing, or at least I did up until my shoulder replacement and few years ago. I like volleyball, Kayaking, biking also.

Q: How often do you play tennis now?

A: Well, up until I ruined my good shoulder I played tennis 3 times a week, now I'm down to twice a week, and volleyball once a week, I also play golf twice a week. I'm pretty happy with my physical condition now thanks to modern medicine.

Brian P. Bradley
Age 62 – Athletic – Skier, Tennis player Upper level & competitive, playing in 4.5 & 5.0 tournaments.
Retired commercial airline pilot
Double hip replacement – April 2000

Q: What was the main reason you decided to get both hips replaced?

A: I was taking my father to the doctor about his hips that were being looked at, and found that there were 10 hip replacements in my family. As far as symptoms, when I was jogging I began to feel a twinge in my hip flexor. I thought it was just maybe a glitch, but then it happened repeatedly. I had X-rays and found I had degeneration and arthritis. It was recommended that I have both hips replaced in the next 2 years, so that's what I did.

Q: When you decided to do it your health insurance in place?

A: Yes I was fully covered by the airline I for which I flew. They had a great insurance plan.

Q: So you decided to have both hips replaced and what was the timetable?

A: I wanted both done at the same time, and my doctor said he would not do both at once, but recommended replacing one and then at least 6 weeks later replace the second one. He wanted to see how the first one worked out, and then he said when I walked in unassisted with no problem, he would do the remaining hip.

Q: How long was your recovery time from the day you had the operation until you were walking with no problem?
A: Well, as I mentioned the first one was 6 weeks, and I was walking without a walker or cane. This qualified me to get the second hip replaced as far as my doctor was concerned. After the second hip was replaced, it was about the same amount of time before I was again walking without any additional support.

Q: What kind of painkiller did they give you to use at home?
A: I remember it was Percocet.

Q: Did you have any trouble getting off the drug once you quit taking it?
A: No not really, I didn't really feel the need to take it after the 3rd or 4th day after I got home, so there wasn't much of a withdrawal effect when I stopped it. I was glad of that because I have heard stories of people having serious withdrawal symptoms from taking the heavier painkillers for some length of time.

Q: How long was it before you could be effective on the tennis court?
A: It took probably another 2 months of easing into moving around, and building myself back up to where I was before the operations.

Q: That was in 2001 it is now 2016, how are your hips doing?
A: Really good, I'm playing a lot of tennis in Atlanta, the tennis Mecca of the U.S. , belong to a great tennis club here, and I am on 3 leagues, and play an average of 5 to 6 matches a week. Although it's a lot of doubles, I can still play singles if I want, the hips are holding up in fine fashion. Having the surgery has alleviated all the joint pain and I feel great, I'm very happy with the results, and feel it was a very wise decision to get the procedure done.

Lee Smoot – Laguna Niguel
Age 65
Waiter – Montage Hotel Laguna Niguel Ca.
Hip replacement & knee operation.

Q: Lee why did you feel you needed a hip replacement?
A: After the X-rays my doctor told me there was no way I could go on being productive in my job as a waiter at this major hotel resort unless I get both hips replaced. I realized he was right because the Rheumatoid Arthritis I had in both hips was totally debilitating and I could hardly walk. I had to walk like I was on stilts, rocking back and forth.

Q: What did you decide to do?
A: I said “Let’s go for it” and I was scheduled for surgery “Sometime” in the next 4 months.
When my wife heard the news that it was 4 months before I was to get the surgery, she was very concerned, and said that was not acceptable. She called the surgeon back and told him that I couldn’t last 4 months being in the condition I was in. The Doctor called me back in a week and said that there was a cancelation and I could get the first hip done in about 30 days. This was great news and I was scheduled for surgery at that time. The surgery went well and I was laying there in my bed the day after and they came in to my room and said “It’s time to get up and do some walking”. I did get out of bed, used the walker they

gave me and did 3 “Laps” around the floor I was staying on.

Q: What did you think about attempting to walk so soon?
A: I thought that it was totally amazing that I could actually be walking so soon after my surgery, but also, it’s amazing what a few pain pills can do for you.

Q: When did your have your second hip replaced?
A: My surgeon scheduled my next hip replacement for 45 days in the future, so I knew what to expect and there were no surprises, so it was much the same experience as the first operation.

Now 2 years later I have a knee problem because I have worn out a lot of the cartridge in my right knee and need some “Work” done on it to give me the mobility I need to do my job.
They gave me the “Gel” injections and they seem to help but it’s not like it’s a “Cure-all” for my problem. It only lasts a few months and then it’s back to same ‘ole same ‘ole, but the hips are doing fine.

Timothy McPherson Age 71
Laguna Niguel, Ca.
13 Surgeries – 2 Knee & Hip Replacements, shoulder reconstruction, elbow surgery.

Q: What was the main factor in your deciding to get a total knee replacement?
A: Well I've had 13 surgeries due to sports injuries, and the like. One was for a shoulder separation, then both knees and hips, to repair the damaged cartilage, and a year ago both knees replaced. In general it was the level of pain on the knees to just walk. I've done sports all my life and that results in an exceeding level of pressure on all your joints. Like they say, "It's not your age, it's the mileage." Just the level of pain to go about my daily activities is what makes you want to correct it with whatever method you feel will do the job.

Q: What kind of sports were you in to?
A: Well, I did quite a few, tennis, skiing, volleyball, and baseball. That is what probably gave my elbow a big problem as a pitcher in an A level baseball league.

Q: How long were you in the hospital?
A: Just 2 days for the knees and hips, it's wonderful the way they can do these replacements and get you walking in just a day or two. I was really surprise the first time with the knee replacement; they had me up and using a walker

strolling down the hall of the hospital at the beginning of the second day.

Q: What did they give you for the pain in the initial days of recovery?
A: I think it was Oxycodone or some other opioid type of painkiller. It seemed to do the job, but there wasn't a lot of pain so to speak. I really didn't take a lot of the pills in the first month, after that I felt ok without taking anything at all. Some people, from what I understand have more of a problem with pain, but I've never been one of them, so I didn't rely a lot of the painkillers, I don't like to take any more meds than totally necessary if I don't have to.

Q: Were there any withdrawal symptoms when you quit taking the Oxycodone?
A: No, not really, I didn't take them as much as the prescription recommended, and when I quit taking them I did it in a controlled manner like the instructions said, by tapering off instead of just quitting overnight.

Q: How long did it take you to be able to resume your regular sports activities after the surgery?
A: Well, they told me to wait 3 months before putting any real pressure on the knee (or later the hip when I had it replaced) , but I was out there just rallying with one of my friends on the tennis court at the end of the second month. They told me

to take it easy and let pain be the determining factor on how much pressure I could put on the knee (and hip) so that's what I did. Then there is the factor of how your muscles have weakened because of non-use for the past couple of months. I started my therapy after about the second week after surgery, going to the gym and working with a professional therapist. It's funny how time goes so slow when you want things to happen with your body's healing, and reconstruction, but eventually it begins to come around again. The trouble is, the older you get, the slower it bounces back from not being used in an athletic sense.

Q: So, how long has it been since your most recent replacement?

A: It's been 2 years, and I'm doing as good as I could expect for a person of my age, which is way above the average 71 year old. Most of the people my age just don't have that active a lifestyle, and are overweight, have heart problems, or some other physical problems and I want to scream at them saying, "Get out there and do something physical!" But it's their life and their problem if they want to be a couch potato, I'm just glad I'm me and do what I do, and I feel great and recommend getting yourself "Fixed up" no matter what the problem is, if it can be fixed. You've only got one life and one body so take care of it!

Lisa Soule
Age 55
Long Beach Ca.
Hip Replacement - 2006

Well, I had osteoarthritis and I couldn't even walk out to get the mail, not to mention walk my dog or do most anything that a normal person does when it involves movement on your feet. It just hurt terribly and my world was just closing up, I just didn't want to walk any more than I had to.

Q: Did you take some kind of pain meds for this?
A: Before I had the surgery, they put me on an anti-inflammatory, and it really didn't make things better, I realized something was going to have to be done to improve my situation.

Q: How long were you in the hospital?
A: I went home on the 3rd day after the surgery. They had me doing a little walking with a walker after the first day, and there was a little pain, but I was still doped up from the pain meds they were giving me through my arm.

Q: What kind of painkillers did they give you to take home when you left?
A: I believe it was one of opioids like Percocet, yes that was it.

Q: Was that effective for the pain.
A: Yes, it seemed to dull the pain, but at the same time I felt sluggish, and kind of doped up. I didn't like that, but it was better than the pain I suppose.

Q: How long did you take it?
A: Just for about 2 weeks, if the pain got more than I wanted to endure. I know how addicting those drugs can be, so I wanted to stay clean as much as I could.

Q: How long were you laid up from doing just your regular activities?
A: Well, my husband took care of me for a couple of weeks, and he went to Europe with our children, and then my sister came a stayed with me for a couple of more weeks. So I'd say for about 3 and half or four weeks. Part of that time I was up and moving around, using a walker.

Q: Did you start using a cane after the walker?
A: Yes, I did use a cane for a little bit, but it seemed to get better very quickly. I think after going through the experience, it would really be necessary to have someone to take care of you as a live-in care giver, because otherwise it would really be greatly inconvenient to do simple tasks, and functions without them. After that initial period of about 2 to 3 weeks, then you begin to be able to do things for yourself in a more convenient manner and you need less help.

Harry Morales – 69 – Tennis player, skier, golfer
Laguna Ca. merchant
Laguna Ca.
Knee Replacement

Q: What prompted you to get a total knee replacement?
A: Pain while putting any pressure on the joint. I enjoy playing tennis on an upper level, and it got to a point where I just couldn't run at first, then take even a few steps in the direction I wanted. I was diagnosed as having arthritic joints and very little cartilage left in my knee joint. I was taking the Glucosamine, but that didn't seem to do much good, so I realized there was only one option, get it done.

Q: What kind of sports if any were you into.
A: Although I enjoy skiing, volleyball, and golf, my main sport I enjoy is tennis. I've been playing competitive for 25 years, and really enjoy the sport a lot, so when my knee began giving me a problem I was really disappointed in that it seriously prevented me from being competitive with the people I was used to playing with.

Q: How long were you in the hospital?
A: Just 2 and a half days. I came home on the 3rd day. The doctor was great, and the surgery went very well, they did a great job of stitching me up, you can hardly see any kind of a scar.

Q: After the hospital morphine what did they give you for pain to take home with you?
A: I think it was called Norco, and I didn't really have that much pain, so in an effort not to use prescription pain meds, I began taking Tylenol. That seem to be enough to help the pain, and I felt better about the fact that I was not on a stronger pain medication.

Q: So then there probably not a lot of withdrawal symptoms were there?
A: No, and from what I hear, that's a major problem for a lot of people that have taken the heavier painkillers, like Norco, Oxycodone, and Percocet. I'm glad I could handle the rehab with only an over-the-counter painkiller.

Q: How soon did they get you up and moving around?
A: On the second day I was doing laps up and down the hospital hallway using a walker. I felt pretty good, had a small amount of pain, but everything felt good. I was putting most of the pressure on the walker at first, but then as I got more confidence with my new knee, I began to put more pressure on it.

Q: How long was it before you could begin to resume your regular "Non-athletic" activities like walking, driving etc.
A: It was about 2 weeks after I got home from the hospital. I was using a cane for the first 4 or 5 days

to just take a little bit of the weight off of the knee, and then I began to feel confident enough to put a normal amount of pressure on the leg. In another week I was climbing stairs without much trouble and getting dressed and undressed by myself easily. It's pretty difficult to get pants on by yourself when you can't bend your leg very well.

Q: How about driving your vehicle, when did you feel it was safe to resume operation.
A: Well, since I was not taking any of the prescription pain meds to affect my reactions, and since it was my left knee which is inactive using an automatic transmission, I started driving again after about the 3rd week. The main challenge was getting in an out of my truck which sits about 2 feet off the ground, but it all worked out fine.

Q: How long was it before you could resume an exercise pattern putting pressure on your knee.
A: Well, they start your professional therapy in about 3 weeks after surgery, such as trying to develop flexibility of the joint, and building up of the surrounding muscles. After that you begin to do the muscle exercises, and that takes a while, because those muscles have been inactive for quite a while, and the older you are, the longer it takes to get them back to their former strength.

Q: When did you start to resume your favorite sport?

A: Well, they tell you to wait at least 3 months before putting any "Athletic" pressure on the joint, but I was out on the tennis court after about 2 months, 2 weeks, and I felt pretty good to move around. I didn't try any crazy stuff like actually running and stopping, but I was amazed at the fact I could actually put SOME weight on my new knee, and take a couple of steps in the right direction.

Q: How long has it been now since the operation?
A: It's been approximately a year, and I am moving as well as I ever have. It's really great to be able to get back into the game of tennis and be competitive again.

Q: What would you say to someone that was in your situation before the surgery?
A: I am so glad I had this done, I would recommend that if someone is in the same situation of pain with their knee or even hip, that they don't wait another day without seeking help and consultation on getting this procedure done. Life is too short to go through it with a problem like this. And the older you get the harder it is on you.

Chapter 10
What does it all mean?

Now that you've hopefully got more information about these procedures than you did before reading this, what are you going to do about it?

There are two kinds of people in the world, one type gravitates toward the positive, and the other type runs away from the negative. Meaning that it is more important to the first group to see what's good about something and try to achieve that end because of positive results that may be attained. The other group feels it is more important to pick the variable that will insulate them from what will hurt them or protect them from a negative occurrence. With these people it's more important to be protected from negative experiences, than to achieve positive ones.

In the end they may make the same choice, but for different reasons. You have to evaluate your situation from one of those two vantage points. Some people like myself, want to get a joint replacement because of how it will improve their abilities in their favorite sport, others feel that they need it to keep them from the pain they feel when doing daily activities. For some people the decision is made for them, in that they have no choice, it's cane, crutches, or a wheelchair and that's the end of it.

If you are in the grey area of deciding on whether to have the procedure done or not and it is hard for you to come to that decision, then take a tip from everyone who contributed to this book. They all seem to have one common realization in their post-operation evaluation. “I should have done it sooner” or “My life is so much better now.”

At the close if this writing I am in my 16th week of post-operation, and have been on the tennis court for about 4 weeks, each week getting better and more mobile. I can tell you that the joy of being able to do something I really love, and to be competitive again, and do “Battle” with my friends in that competitive area, is a wonderful feeling.

It was such a great feeling on that first day back on the court just rallying hitting a few shots in practice. I had this great mental exhilaration the first time someone hit me a high lob. I had to go back about 4 steps to get into position, and as I was doing that, in putting weight on my “New” knee, I was so amazed that it took the weight without pain, that the conscious thought shot through my mind that actually said, “Oh ya, now that’s what I’m talking about, I’m back!” I felt like I won the lottery, pulled King Arthur’s sword from the stone, caught the winning Super Bowl pass…just for a few seconds. I wouldn’t trade that for anything in the world, and neither will you, when you come back to the world of “Mobil without pain”. So in an effort to help your decision making process, I will make this suggestion that may sound overly simple, it’s like I’ve said in all my books and articles…

JUST DO IT!

And the best of luck

Roger W. Breterntiz CCht.

Other publications by this author:

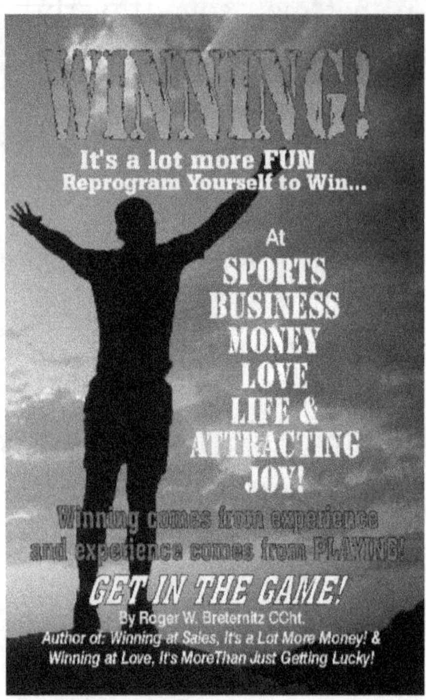
WINNING!
It's a lot more FUN
Reprogram Yourself to Win...
At
SPORTS
BUSINESS
MONEY
LOVE
LIFE &
ATTRACTING
JOY!
Winning comes from experience
and experience comes from PLAYING!
GET IN THE GAME!
By Roger W. Breternitz CCht.
Author of: Winning at Sales, It's a Lot More Money! &
Winning at Love, It's MoreThan Just Getting Lucky!

Yes it's a lot more fun when you win. Someone said, "It doesn't matter if you win or lose...until you lose! Now that's real truth.

This is a 350 page collection of winning strategies, ideas, articles and formulas to make you a winner in every phase of your life. Written by Roger W. Breternitz CCht. it contains secrets of the world champions, insights about turning your desires in to actual reality, and converting ideas into deposits for your bank account, along with just how to attract joy in your life.

To sum it up: It's how your mental state and thoughts affect your physical world and draw to you the things you WANT or DON'T want.

This is a book created from a wealth of 37 years of professional business sales and management, being a professional musician/band leader, tennis and ski instructor, engineering designer, writer for a national sports magazine, and hypnotherapist with 27 years experience in helping people restructure, and motivate their lives.
Available at Amazon.com

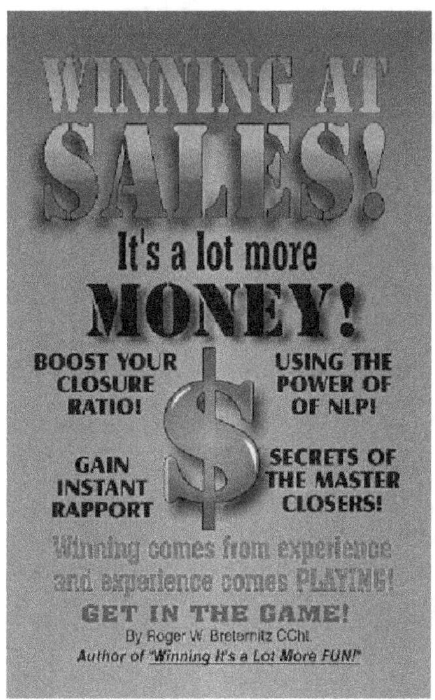
WINNING AT
SALES!
It's a lot more
MONEY!
BOOST YOUR CLOSURE RATIO!
USING THE POWER OF OF NLP!
GAIN INSTANT RAPPORT
SECRETS OF THE MASTER CLOSERS!
Winning comes from experience and experience comes PLAYING!
GET IN THE GAME!
By Roger W. Breternitz CCht.
Author of "Winning It's a Lot More FUN!"

It has been said that over 90% of people making their living in sales, have never read ONE book on the art of selling. If you are one of these people THIS is the one book to read!! If you are now in sales or want to get into sales, and realize you don't know everything there is to know about how to create rapport, instill confidence, and close more business, then you really need this book! It contains the secrets of Neuro-Linguist Programming, embedded commands, analog marking, matching, mirroring and pacing, eye blink technique, and many other little known "Deal closing" concepts only known by the few upper level "Master closers". This is a boiled down and simplified collective of over 25 years experience and 16different sales training programs from major corporations. It provides you with powerful information and techniques that you can take out an use instantly, turning your efforts and your phone into a cash cow like never before. So don't wait until your company tells you that you need to "Meet or exceed quota" to keep your desk, start WINNING AT SALES today, it's a lot money! Available at Amazon.com

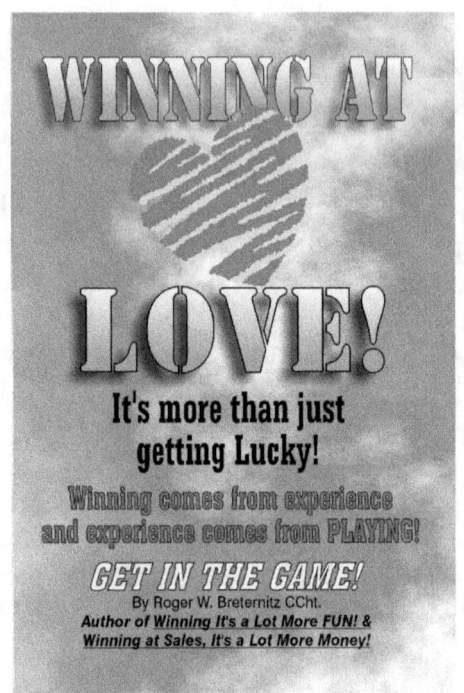

It's more than just
getting Lucky!
Winning comes from experience

GET IN THE GAME!

There have been hundreds of books out there written that claim to guide you in how to attract the opposite sex, but very few of them if any, give you actual *tools* to do just that. What your inner mind believes, controls what your outward behavior demonstrates. "Winning at Love" is a step-by-step instructional manual showing you how to reprogram your inner mind that WILL alter your outward behavior to make you more attractive to those "Just right" members of the opposite sex. It focuses on how to build self-confidence, and uses the practice of Neuro-Linguistic Programming to implant suggestions and get the desired responses from anyone you meet, and it is written with both men and women in mind. Get Winning at Love NOW, and in 30 days or less, attract that person you've been looking for, and recognize them when they come along.
Available at Amazon.com

WEB SITE

http://www.awinnersway.com

Everything you have in life, the people you know, your job, the person you're married to or cling to, is a result of your belief system. A Winners Way is a site that provides the highest quality DVSs and CDs for the purpose of altering this belief system for the positive, to bring your life the results you want, and it's guaranteed.

Thoughts are things! If you want to change what you have, and live on a higher level...change what you think, and how you think. Just because you're checking out this book in the first place says you either know the power of the sub-conscious, or have become interested in the power of subliminal change, relaxation reprogramming, and or the science of mental reprogramming. Here's your chance to find out what it's all about, and take the first step in a new and rewarding journey toward a better, stronger, higher thinking YOU!
Some of the subjects on CD are:

- Pain Anesthesia
- Lose Weight
- Quit Smoking
- Stress Management
- Athletic Proficiency
- Don't Drink & Drive
- Subliminal Seduction
- Sales Power Persuasion
- Stuttering Solved
- Custom created CD's – Any subject

Surgery Documentation/Workbook

Below you can create a "Diary" type of documentation, where you can write your perceptions and experiences of your surgery, which will give you a retrospective look at how it all went, what your feelings were, and what you should have done better or did well and document the dates and time of the event for future use such as insurance payments co-payments and more.

Initial consultation (Date)________________________

Doctor Name ________________________________

Results ____________________________________

Initial Screening Date__________________________

Results ____________________________________

Surgery date set as __________________________

Time ______________________________________

Hospital Stay:

1st Day - Activities (Meals, pain level, walking if any, tests etc.)

____

____

____

2nd Day

____

____

____

3rd Day

____

____

____

DRUGS:

Pain medication / Dosage__________________________________

How many weeks taken __________________________________

Experiences ____

THERAPY:

Started on ____

Therapist ____

Times per week ______________________________________

Results & Progress ____________________________________

Post opp experiences (reactions to drugs & withdrawals recuperations

____

____

____

____

____

____

____

____

____

INSURANCE INFORMATION:

Name of insurer: ____

Type of Plan ____

Policy Number ______________________________________

Co-Pay for this procedure ________________________________

Contact info at insurance co. ______________________________

Date Paid co-pay ______________________________________

Miscellaneous data:

____

____

____

____

____

____

____

____

About the Author

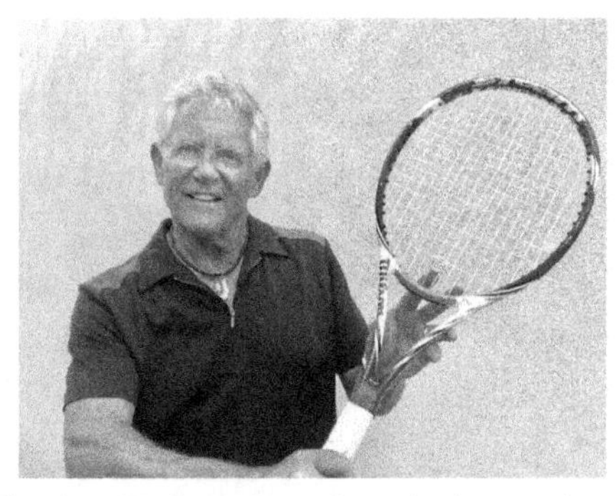

Roger W. Breternitz – CCht. Hypnotherapist, Salesman, Author, Tennis Pro, Trainer A graduate of Illinois State University with a degree in Education and Southern Illinois University in design and graphics, he makes his home in Laguna Niguel, California. With certifications in Clinical Hypnotherapy and Neuro Linguistic Programming, he is now currently presenting lectures and seminars on the art of sales and quality communication for corporations and sales organizations wanting to improve their profit margin and inter-office harmony. In his book "Winning it's a lot more fun!" he draws on his experience in being a tennis teaching pro, high school tennis coach, world class archer, top level trap shooter, and studying many champions and sports gurus on how the mind works to make you a winner in sports as well as life in general, and how some people program it to do just the opposite. The Knee / Hip Replacement book was created to help those of you who are trying to decide what to do about your ageing joints and possible limited mobility. He hopes it has in some way given you a little insight as to what you may experience if you decide to have the procedure. You may find some answers to even the "Unasked" questions about attracting more positive results in your life on his web site http://www.awinnersway.com

About the Author

www.ingramcontent.com/pod-product-compliance
Lightning Source LLC
Chambersburg PA
CBHW060357190526
45169CB00002B/644